Your Transplant Adventure!

A Kid's Guide to Organ Transplant

D1598619

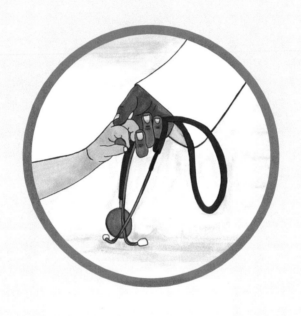

Your Transplant Adventure!

A Kid's Guide to Organ Transplant

Matt Butler, LMSW

Tanya Smith, LMSW

Edited by Stacy Brand
University of Michigan Transplant Center
Michigan Medicine

Illustrations by Melissa Mueller

Book design by Kevin Woodland
Health Information Technology & Services
Michigan Medicine

Produced by Health Information Technology & Services,
Michigan Medicine

Published by Michigan Publishing
University of Michigan Library

Rev. 1 / July, 2018

ISBN: 978-1-60785-497-5 (print)
ISBN: 978-1-60785-498-2 (ebook)

DEDICATION

We dedicate this book to all of the children who have received a transplant, and those who are still waiting for their second chance at life. We created this book to give children and their families something to help make them more at ease with the transplant process and to let them know that they are not alone. We hope you find the information in this book helpful as a means of talking openly about transplantation with your children.

ACKNOWLEDGMENTS

*We would like to thank the following
individuals for their support:*

John Magee, MD
Jeremiah and Claire Turcotte
Professor of Transplant Surgery,
Professor of Internal Medicine and Pediatrics,
and University of Michigan Transplant
Center Director, Michigan Medicine

Helen Costis, MHSA
University of Michigan Transplant Center
Director of Operations, Michigan Medicine

Drs. Emily Fredericks and Melissa Cousino
Pediatric Transplant Psychologists, Michigan
Medicine, for their review of the content of this book

Stacy Brand, MBA
University of Michigan Transplant Center
Outreach Manager, Michigan Medicine,
for her coordination and communication role
in bringing this book to reality

Funding for this publication was made possible
by the University of Michigan Transplant Center.

What is a transplant?

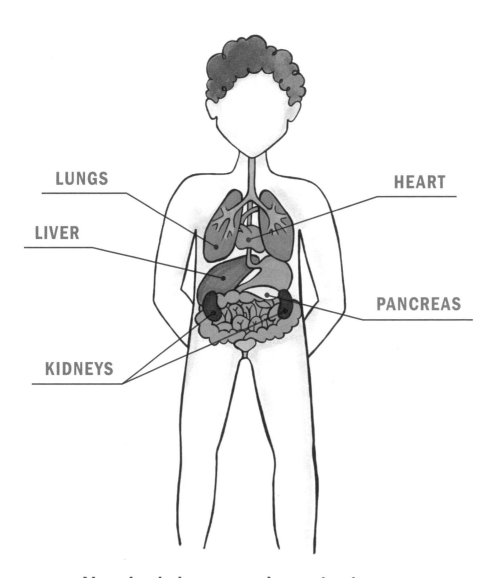

LUNGS

HEART

LIVER

PANCREAS

KIDNEYS

Your body has many important organs inside. Sometimes, one or more organs can be sick. A transplant replaces the sick organ with a healthy one.

What kind of transplant do I need?

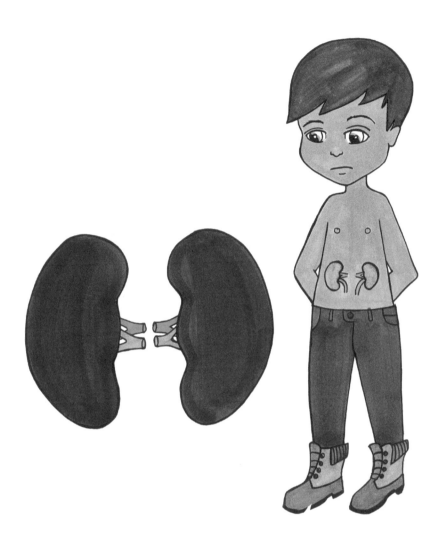

There are other kids like you who need organ transplants. Some kids need more than one kind of transplant and others need only one. This boy needs a kidney transplant.

Where will my new organ come from?

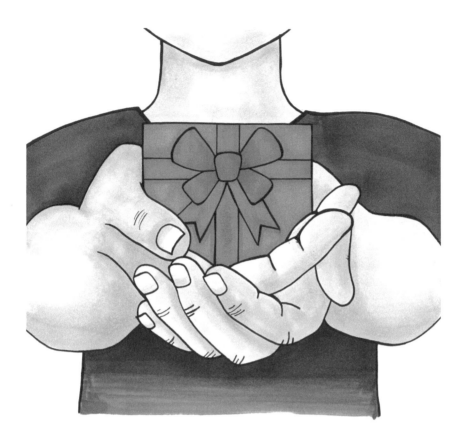

New organs come from a donor. A donor
could be someone who is alive who gives
all or part of an organ to you. An organ
may also come from someone who died.
Their family decided to give their organs
to help someone else.

How will I know when it's time for my transplant?

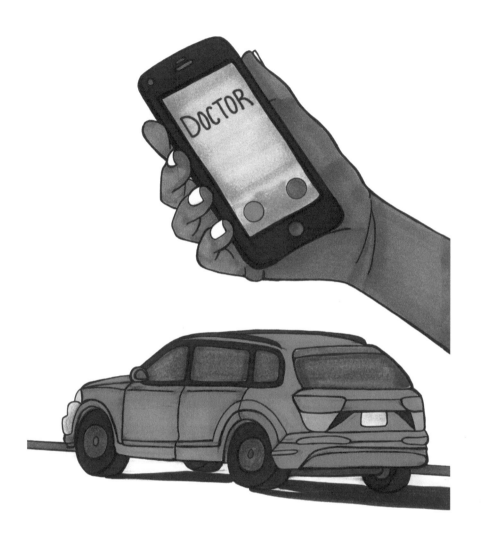

A doctor or nurse will call your family to tell them there is an organ ready for you.

What happens next?

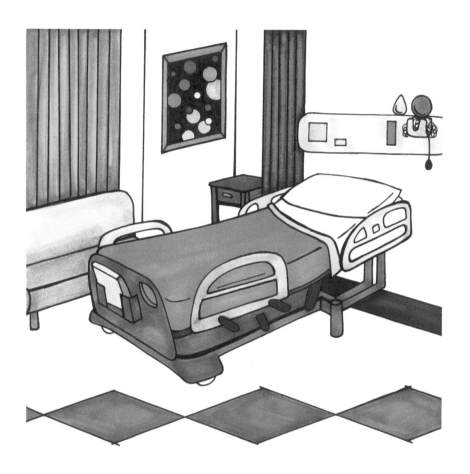

If you are at home, you and your family will come to the hospital to get ready for surgery. If you are in the hospital already, the doctors and nurses will help you get ready for the operation. Transplant surgery is when the doctors put in your new organ.

What will the surgery be like?

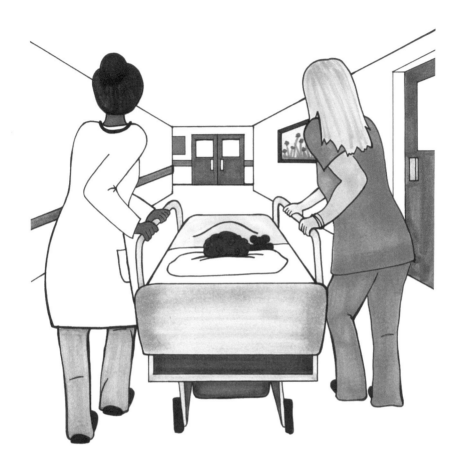

Doctors and nurses will give you medicine
to help you take a nap. You will sleep
through the whole surgery. The doctors
and nurses wake you up in a hospital room
with your family when the surgery is over.

will it hurt?

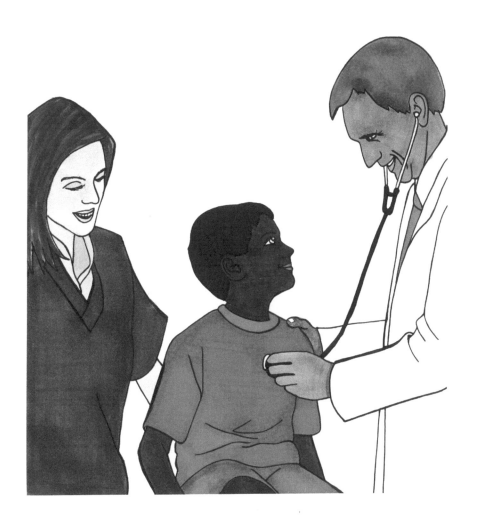

Sometimes having surgery does hurt.
There are many things that will help you feel
better—medicine, watching your favorite
movie, or playing a game. Your doctors and
nurses are here to help and make sure you
feel better as fast as you can!

Will I have stitches or a scar?

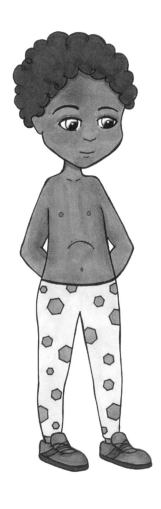 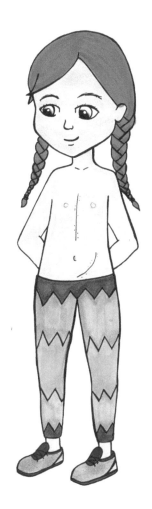

Your doctor will use stitches or a special kind of glue to help your body heal from the surgery. After the stitches come out, you will have a scar. This will always remind you of how brave you were!

What do I need to do to keep my new organ healthy?

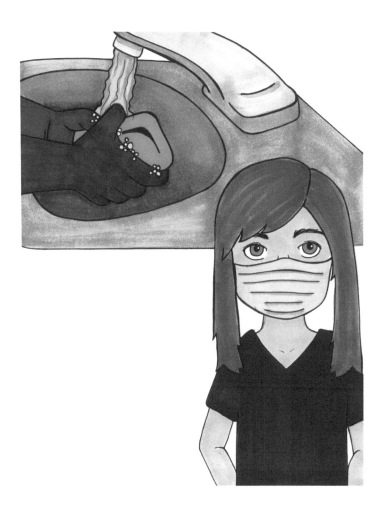

After your transplant, you will need to protect your body from germs. You will need to wear a mask for a while when you leave your house. It will also be very important to wash your hands.

Will I take medicine?

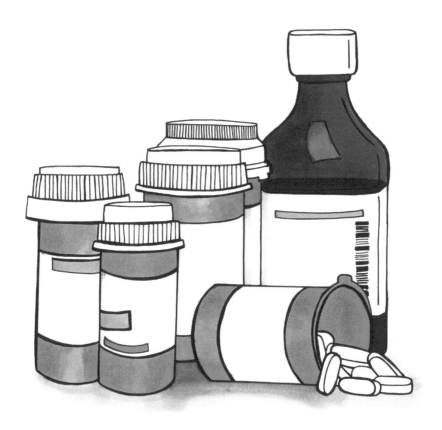

After your transplant, you will have
new medicines that you will take
every day. Sometimes they are
liquid and sometimes they are pills.

Will I still have to come to the hospital?

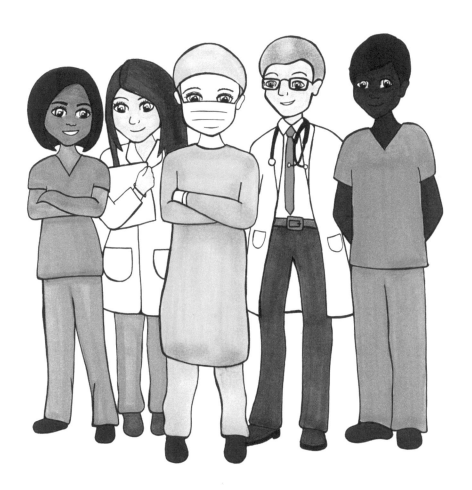

You will always need to see a doctor for your new transplant. At first you will need to see a doctor every week, but eventually you will only need to see a doctor a few times a year.

Will I be able to go back to school?

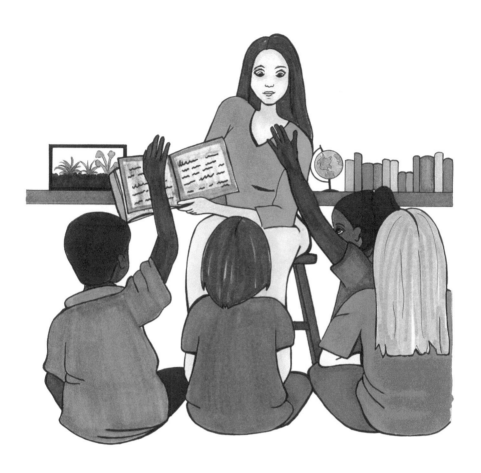

You will need to stay home from
school for a few weeks after having your
transplant. Your doctor and nurses
will let you know when you are ready
to go back to school again.

How will I feel after my transplant?

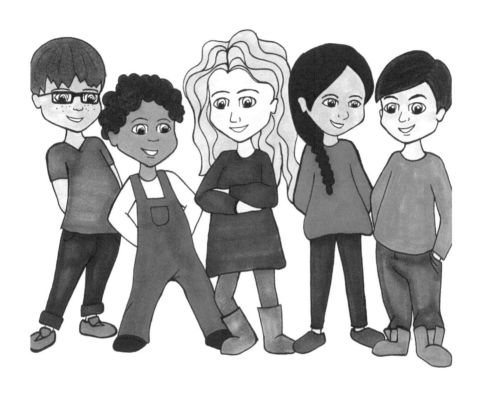

After transplant, you should start to
feel better and have more energy to play.
Remember, you are never alone.
There are other kids just like you
who have had transplants, too!

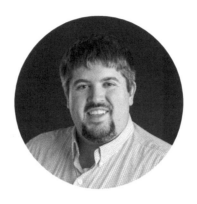

Matt Butler, co-author

Matt Butler, LMSW, is a Senior Clinical Social Worker in Nephrology and Kidney Transplant since 2012. Matt graduated with a Masters in Social Work from the University of Michigan School of Social Work in 2011. He was Chair of the Michigan Council of Nephrology Social Workers from 2016-2017 and has been involved in this organization since 2012. Matt was named as the National Kidney Foundation Pediatric Nephrology Social Worker of the Year in 2017. He was nominated for the University of Michigan Transplant Center Employee of the Year in 2014. Matt is an advocate for children with kidney disease, and he is dedicated to improving the lives of each of his patients through his work. Matt lives in Michigan with his wife and enjoys spending time with his family.

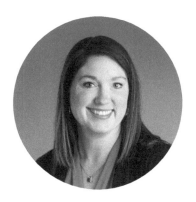

Tanya Smith, co-author

Tanya Smith, LMSW, is a Senior Clinical Social Worker in Pediatric Liver Transplant since 2009. Tanya graduated with a Masters in Social Work from the University of Michigan School of Social Work in 2007. She was nominated for the 2018 Beverly Jean Howard Award for Excellence in Social Work at Michigan Medicine. She has participated in research efforts at Michigan Medicine in the field of pediatric liver transplant, is actively engaged in the development and provision of patient education, and enjoys serving as a champion for transplant patients and their families. She has spent time volunteering as a counselor at Camp Michitanki, a summer camp program for solid organ transplant recipients. Tanya lives in Michigan with her husband and their two daughters.

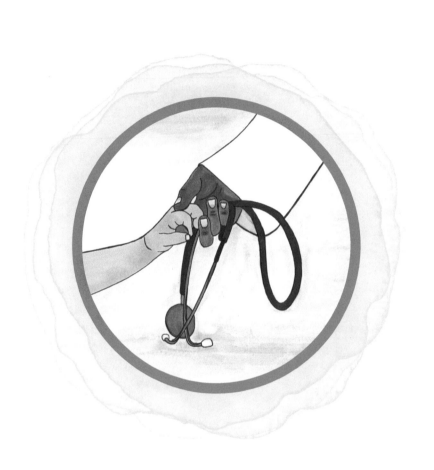

CPSIA information can be obtained
at www.ICGtesting.com
Printed in the USA
LVHW071623110920
665712LV00001B/4

* 9 7 8 1 6 0 7 8 5 4 9 7 5 *